THE HEALING ANGEL

Cornelius O. Barlascini

For Laura and Louis, to help them understand

*The Institute for the Study of the History of Medicine
provided assistance with research as well specific medical*

Footnotes are always a problem.

Very few people want to go through 100 citations.

The citations are embedded within the text.

What I have done here is cite only quotations, unique observations.

CONTENTS

AN ANGELIC ALLEGORY

I ask the reader to indulge the author's macroscopic view of the universe so that we can go from the general to the particular. To understand man, we must start with all that is in heaven, earth, and hell. We will finish with one doctor and one patient.

We need to define several words, giving them very specific meanings. Positive in this book means information free of ethical or moral content. Ethics refer to particular normative statements based on profession, tribe, culture, or nationality. Moral statements refer to divine fiats. Normative statements are those that contain a judgment, concerning any relationship of objects that cannot be directly measured or any assertion based on any supposition or intuition. Positive statements: wild boars are mammals; wild boars usually have four legs; wild boars eat both plant and animal life. Normative statements: it must have been a wild boar that wrecked my garden last night. Wild boars are God's agents of retribution; they wrecked my garden because I am a sinner. The reader will find that I label my normative statements quite clearly. He (or she, I am using the masculine pronoun to represent all humans) will find that evolution is a normative word. It carries judgments within itself. Natural selection and adaptation are more likely to be positive words. These latter two words may describe a particular situation in objective matter. The only normative aspect of these terms is the presumption that the survival and reproduction of a particular species in a particular time and place is a good thing. That's the normative baggage of natural selection and adaptation. As the reader will see, it is difficult to make completely positive statements. Of course, there are tautologies. God exists, or He does not. Statements about existence are always positive. It is raining or not. Statements about attributes may be either positive or normative. Existence is not an attribute; it is that "object" to which attributes are ascribed.

Now we have to move to the basic assumption: you and I exist in a real world. Life is not a dream; we are not creatures held by strings in the hands of some mysterious puppet master. We must also concede that there are parameters which are predetermined by our genes, by the circumstances of our birth, by history itself, and by the limitations of the human body. We cannot fly by flapping our arms. We cannot travel back and forward in time. However, we get to make some choices. We make a major choice which changes the way we perceive the world: invisible atoms, molecules, and cells or five elements (earth, air, fire, ether, and water). We can decide if there is a

God, more than one, or none. We can decide if death is the end or merely a new beginning. Finally, there are two fundamental decisions that are more difficult to make. The first regards a proposition that seems silly: "you can't put your foot in the same stream twice". In other words, each moment in life is unique. The second concerns a theory that few of us ever consider: there is a hemisphere of sunlight that is common to all of us and is subject to the laws of science. There is another hemisphere, a place of darkness, which is unique to each individual, and it is the world of dreams, souls, and the unconscious mind. There exists a single world with two hemispheres. Like the moon, the dark side is hidden, but real.

These two hemispheres are one and the same, as are the faces of a single coin. As a matter of fact, this was a famous coin. It was the coin that the Pharisees gave to Jesus; they wanted to trick him into either blasphemy or treason. Jesus looked at the coin with its portrait of the paranoid, perverted Tiberius and understood that there was one answer to this question. Is it proper to pay taxes to the emperor? Jesus knew another answer that changed the nature of the question. It was an answer that cut like the blades of hundred swords: "render unto to Caesar what is Caesar's". This is not solely a theological response; it is also a philosophical response: whatever is evil cannot produce good. The product of evil is never good. Return evil to its origin without touching it.

The author is going to make up a little story. In the beginning God was not alone. He had created seven archangels before time began. There was Gabriel who was supposed to announce great events to mankind. He also wrestled with Jacob. The hip injury was a reminder that the patriarch was human and not divine. Certainly, it was a painful lesson. However, Jacob had to realize that even the father of the Twelve Tribes was human. Raphael helped Jacob after the combat. This angel was the friend of the sick; he made sure that Jacob was not disabled after the contest. This is not in the Bible because Raphael had the dignity of the true physician; he insisted on confidentiality.

And then there was Michael; he was the saddest of all the angels. He was consumed with worry that "the absence of good" would consume all Creation. He was the first to question God, endless demands concerning morality. He got God to admit that good could produce evil, and that evil could never produce good fruits. This is another fundamental rule of philosophy and theology.

All these seven angels had free will. Man revered these three angels; however, the other four were not so well known or so well liked. There was an angel called Virtue that fluttered about God's head. His job was to make sure God did nothing wrong. And this was indeed strange because God was supposed to be perfect. What was the use of a nagging conscience for the Almighty? Virtue had been made to satisfy man. He was the greatest angel, commanded all the others; after all, he was the extension of God's mind. For Plato and many others there was a need for God to be perfect, and this was the way to make it so.

Now, the reader must understand that these four angels looked like angels were supposed to look:

white gown, two feathery wings starting at the shoulder ending at the buttocks. The other three were different in appearance.

There was a fly, a big fly, the size of your thumb nail. You could see him, but you had to look for him. Socrates would have called him a gadfly; he had a tiny shirt on which was written Mef. His job was to inspire man to achievement: technological or artistic advances were always positive. He gave no thought to normative considerations; man had free will for those considerations. Maybe God knew man would fail in Eden, so He wanted man to have some help. If that was His plan, it backfired. Man kept choosing evil. The species seemed not to know any better.

Long before man existed, two of the angels turned against God. The first was the angel who seemed to be the ideal of God's beauty. All who saw him in Heaven and on the Earth held him up as the mirror of all beauty. Even God loved him the most; he was a mirror of God's majesty. He was clad in a garment of thousand colors, all different, all beautiful. The light from his face lit all of Heaven. Lucifer was a reflection of God's glory.

Finally, there was another archangel. He was God's butler. He had all the keys to all the gates, to all the store rooms, to all the riches of Heaven. He had no face. In fact, none of his "flesh" was visible. His hands were gloved in white. His hood was white, and no light came from his eyes.

Something happened that God could have not stopped. You would think that God could do anything. However, two things stood in God's path.

The first was that every Archangel had free will and great power. The second was that Virtue rejected our little gadfly; Virtue without Knowledge is defective. That's another axiom. Virtue never believed that anything God made could become evil. You must understand that our gadfly knew only of the past and the present; however, he could calculate the rough probability of every possible consequence (from almost certain to nearly impossible) of future events. For Mef all outcomes were without normative content. He obeyed God in all things, but was morally neutral. In other words he provided the possibilities, but rendered no judgment. God's butler, Beelzebub, pestered Mef to give him the single key that would complete his collection. After billions of years, with tears and shouts, after answering impossible questions, and enduring thousands of humiliating moments, Mef surrendered the key to his personal library. The room was empty. He had disposed of all his manuals. Mef had stuffed all knowledge into his tiny brain. Of course, this brings up another rule. Knowledge cannot be obtained without effort. The keeper of the keys offered the beautiful angel, Lucifer, all the richest and powers of Heaven. All Lucifer had to do was take God's seat. In this way Lucifer learned pride. But this was a special kind of pride. This was the pride of glory unearned. God knew at once of this betrayal. He summoned Michael to cast Satan (no longer the beautiful Lucifer, but a creature resembling a burnt prune) and the Lord of the flies (no longer to Lord of the House, now a ghoulish clown with flies buzzing around him) into Hell. But why flies? That was easy: a mistake, a misprint, **lies, Lord of the lies.** Their descent into hell triggered God's admission to

Michael and exposed Virtue's error. God had created two angels that betrayed Him. Good became evil.

Michael was reluctant to cast out his brothers. Mef spoke: "This dark creature with his clanging keys came to me to ask: What was the most dangerous strategy in the universe? How could God be overthrown? I told the truth. Beelzebub learned that ignorance coupled with unearned pride could overthrow even God. God would have to assume the nature and person of the human to achieve victory. God paid with his endless suffering in the person of Christ or the coming Messiah, (a matter of personal belief that is, of course, outside the scope of this angel). There would be millions of human martyrs and even more "collateral damage. I had no choice: it is my task to tell the truth".

God was angry: "You mean this could happen again?"

Mef replied with great sadness: "I think so. I think, and this is only my opinion, Satan is trying to command Beelzebub. He who served in Heaven now seeks to rule Hell. But he shall not. The force of complete Knowledge is so powerful that once let loose from Heaven it could destroy all creation. Man must have knowledge to be wise and then he may choose the broad highway to perdition or the narrow path to Heaven. I can only tell You the truth. All the greater sins are the product of ignorance. One may be ignorant of God's laws, of how to proceed in one's life. Man had the source of own destruction within him. The weakest of our cadre was the easiest to persuade. The greatest pressure was on the one who was meant to keep order within our universe, our keeper of the keys. Beelzebub will be behind Satan, hiding and controlling him. Satan is but a preening doll controlled by the greatest puppeteer. Knowledge is never freely given. It must be sought and maintained. Knowledge is the hardest thing to obtain and the easiest to lose.

ARISTOTLE AND ANGELS

Aristotle made everything very convenient. It was easy; the earth was the center of the universe. Of course, he got a little help from a certain Greek living in Egypt named Ptolemy. Then it was easy; there were higher animals and lower animals, plants and little stuff that seemed to come out of the mud. Moreover, Aristotle was a tremendous descriptive biologist. Some of the morphology he described was confirmed only in the last century. He was also the only psychologist free of any religious influence until after 1500 AD (at least in the Western world).

But that was just the beginning: people that spoke Greek were fully human as long as they were males. Those that didn't were barbarians. Women were not even worth considering, except as the vessels for the production of other humans. But even that was not enough: Aristotle told you how you should be ruled, what should make you happy, and what you ought to do to be correct in your behavior. Women and barbarians couldn't be happy or ethical because they were not as human as the Greek speaking male.

But there is more. There is Aristotle's physics which we now know to be completely incorrect except for one point: Aristotle had this very neat, compact, and convenient view of God. God in some way initiated the Creation and then went away. At present, we preparing as a species to prove or disprove this positive statement. There are billions of dollars invested in tunnels, metal tubes, and magnets constructed as a giant racetrack for sub-atomic particles. The particle goes round and round; what it produces is supposed to be a long list of answers. This author would have other uses for those funds; however, the particle collider is there, so let us get some answers. Aristotle never told us where God went after being the First Cause. However, there were plenty of Jews, Christians and Muslims to fill in that part. That is the subject of the next chapter. Now we return to Aristotle's version of utopia.

Well, this is really convenient. You could have a male-dominated society served by women and slaves with a set of intellectual and social beliefs that would be unchanging. And the best part was that there was no need for a particular religious view. You could have one, but you did not have to. There were some problems with this view of the world. First, for all those Platonic types, there was not enough mathematics and not enough God. Certainly Aristotle hung on to the classic Greek soul: free will, passion, and intellect. However, he thought that the brain existed to cool the blood and seem to believe that the soul was somewhere in the liver. That was the only explanation he gave; people had been reading livers all over the Mediterranean for at least three thousand years. It was the traditional view. Aristotle was never one to disturb orthodoxy. The gods of Olympus were out of fashion after Alexander the Great found so many other deities during his conquests. However, unlike the more stubborn Hebrew deity, the Olympians never craved a monopoly and never minded going by aliases. That fact gave Aristotle a big advantage over his successors. That's why he last so long. Finally, Aristotle knew when to simplify: one God, no particular name, who stepped out of the way after the moment of creation.

His logic was used almost exclusively until the beginning of the nineteenth century. And it is still valid today. People should study it. Physicians, in particular, should be instructed in this traditional and formal logic. They would make better decisions.

We now realize that the earth moves around the sun, and the sun moves around something else. We have discarded every bit of his physics in favor of a three party system. The first party (classical) includes everything up to the year 1900 and all the technology that has arisen from it. The second party is named

Albert Einstein, and he had major argument with the third party. The third party (quantum mechanics) took Einstein's work mixed up with the work of physicists in the first half of the last century and came up with an all new alphabet signifying particles that are hard to find. There is one such postulated particle that may be considered Aristotle's particle. God is this "graviton". Everything that exists was the result of this particle. Its "progeny" depend on the existence of time, ten other dimensions and probability theory. We will stop a moment here. If the graviton (alias the God particle) is found and the theory of the twenty or so universal constants is verified, then God exists. The positive positions of Aristotle, Plato, and Pythagoras are each vindicated. Atheism would become essentially impossible to defend. Existence is not an attribute. Of course, redemption, salvation, and morality are not considered in this proof. The proof would be scientific and positive. It would be proof of existence. (It would yield many positive statements which would be distorted into various normative propositions of dubious merit. The only correct normative statement would be: "things" are the way they are because "things" are bound by particular rules.)

This is fundamental to medicine's ontology for three reasons. First, this cosmological proof of God's existence says nothing of his attributes and is not normative. That must come from other sources. These sources are known as archetypes. Medicine needs archetypes independent of the Deity.

Second such a demonstration depends upon establishing that the fact (God) is unique. The probability of another entity (chance, luck) establishing the universe would be approaching absolute impossibility. This experiment would answer the ancient query concerning sound, the tree in the empty world, and the receptor of its collapse. No one would have to hear the tree fall because, given the known parameters, we would know when and how it will fall. We could predict its sound as it tumbles. This solves the transmitter and receiver problem by altering the parameters to center on the event itself. This is important because the underlying foundation of medicine is that man can use information and rules to predict likely successive events. We call these processes diagnosis, prognosis, and treatment.

Medicine would be useless if there was no reality. This collider could prove reality exists. That which is real is predictable; its attributes can be defined. After all, what's the use of treating that which is not material (real)? The doctor is a physician, not a *metaphysicist*. Let's return to the present state of knowledge and say a word about composite particles (especially spinning protons seen on magnetic resonance technology).

These composite particles enter our daily lives in medical procedures, nuclear power plants and weapons of war. The outstanding feature of classical physics is that it works for most every situation. The outstanding feature of quantum physics is the principle of uncertainty: The observer changes the observed object. The great exception to this general rule is that once practical applications are developed of quantum mechanics, the uncertainty should be gone. In other words you can rely on the MRI scan of anything: No, you can't. There is always observer error and/or malfunctions in the apparatus. The author is not sure how this uncertainty can be eliminated.

Our next argument is that man cannot be divided into body and soul as mostly expounded by Descartes.

THE MYTH OF THE CARTESIAN MAN

We begin with Darwin (1809-1882). It is easily seen by anyone that evolution is the wrong word to use for the theory of natural selection. Evolution implies progression. The notion of progress through time is completely false. Moreover, natural selection as applied by society has been a rationale for all manner of brutality. Even Thomas Huxley (1825-1895) finally admitted this. Alfred Wallace (1823-1913) had good reason to disavow his previous alliance with Darwin. Wallace was the first scientist to champion "intelligent design" against Darwin. The Darwinian impetus given to rascals such as Herbert Spencer (1820-1903) and Francis Galton (1822-1911) was unstoppable. The justification of mass poverty, human slavery, ethnic cleansing, routine sterilization, and genocide directly arose from Darwin's concept of evolution. Wallace was prudent to remove his name from this fundamentally flawed theory.

Wallace renounced evolution because he felt that there was a profound defect in the theory that he and Darwin had put forth in 1858. Stephen Gould describes Wallace's reason for this retraction.

Wallace recognized that the "higher functions" of man could not be the product of natural selection. Charity, hope, love, self-sacrifice and a host of other abstract nouns could not have resulted from natural section. The notion that such attributes were always present in the genome is an unproven hypothesis, useless to either champions of evolution or intelligent design. Darwin and Wallace's theory depended on the proposition the all change (mutation) comes from the necessity of the moment. What creature would need such complex behaviors in the jungle? The span of human history is too short for such genetic alterations. Wallace's words: "It would imply that to produce the living soul in the marvelous and glorious body of man -- man with his faculties, his aspirations, his powers for good and evil – that this was an easy matter which could be brought about anywhere, in any world." This would violate the basic tenet of natural selection: change occurs over generations and its success is solely based on need. Wallace continues: "It (natural selection) would imply that man is an animal and nothing more, is of no importance in the universe, needed no great preparations for his advent, only, perhaps, a second-rate demon, and a third or fourth-rate earth". This is the concluding passage of *Man's Place in the Universe* (1903). Wallace postulated a universe limited in size with the creation of the earth as its central contingent purpose and the perfection of man as its final and supreme goal. Clearly this cosmology is false.

So how did all this normative material get into the human brain? Here enters one Johann Gottlieb Fichte (1764-1814), a poor boy whose brilliance provided a scholarship to study theology. For reasons that are still mysterious, Fichte's name and preface were omitted from the first edition of *An Attempt at a Critique of all Revelation* (1792), and thus the book, which displayed an extensive and subtle appreciation of Kant's thought, was taken to be the work of Kant himself. Once it became known that Fichte was the author, he could hardly be taken lightly. **For Fichte, any alleged Revelation of God's activity in the world should pass a moral test: namely, no immoral command or action, i.e., nothing that violates the moral law, can be attributed to Him.** My opinion is that this "rule" is true for only normative assertions, archetypes that I will call paradigms; the dogmatic archetypes may be judged immoral or moral or amoral. It does not matter. These latter sets of statements are positive. Moral judgments when acting within archetypes are irrelevant. This is of supreme importance in medicine. For example, an inexpensive antibiotic is no less moral than an expensive one. The decision to substitute Coumadin (well-known as a rat poison) for aspirin in atrial fibrillation is not a normative consideration. The physician cannot know the future implications (i.e., the hope for a longer, better life). For that one must call an astrologer or a homeopathic practitioner.

Dementia is an interesting word; it has the classical root *mente*. So, where is this *mente*? Where is this *mind*? There are two parts to every human. There are the parts internal to him, including the soul. We will shortly provide the anatomy and physiology of this neurological structure. There are also three parts that are external to the individual. One has a demographic (social) identity; one has a personality which is mostly expressed by one's comportment, and a set of thoughts which are expressed externally. This last aspect is the mind. The mind and the intellect are not identical. They have a correspondence; however, the intellect is part of the soul. It is intrinsic to the brain. The famous maker of triangles, Pythagoras, also had time to outline the anatomy of the soul. The soul had three parts according to Pythagoras. There was the intellect. There was also passion. These were described as horses, each pulling in a different direction. There was a fellow in his chariot trying to command these two beasts called the Will. This description was made famous by Plato. We skip forward about twenty-three centuries to Schopenhauer. Things were much simpler. Passion was not one desire but thousands of desires, each person had the same desires with slight variation within each one. There was the passion to eat; there was a sexual desire. William James postulated that there was a desire that Plato, Aquinas, and Spinoza among many others believed existed. This passion was belief itself; William James called this "the will to believe". You might believe in your lover, your children potential, your country's nationalistic goals... But James was talking about believing in God. Unfortunately, your lover can betray you with another; your country may have evil designs. But God is always perfect. He is always perfect and will be so forever. According to Fitche, God communicates with us through shared revelation. So the Cartesian man is not necessary. We have a tiny neuron that is the will to believe. All of God's information enters through our senses. If one does not believe in God, simply substitute either universal unconscious or cross-cultural archetypes. So what are these imposed positive archetypes? James Joyce uses linguistic terms which describe the medium and the messages of these divine intrusions. As always there are layers and layers of meaning in his "simple" complaint:

The language in which we are speaking is his before it is mine. How different are the words HOME, CHRIST, ALE, MASTER, on his lips and on mine! I cannot speak or write these words without unrest of spirit. His language, so familiar and so foreign, will always be for me an acquired speech. I have not made or accepted its words. My voice holds them at bay. My soul frets in the shadow of his language. *Portrait of the Artist*, James Joyce 1914-1917, chapter 5

GOD'S LANGUAGE OR THE CROSS CULTURAL UNIVERSALS WILL ALWAYS BE AN ACQUIRED SPEECH, A LANGUAGE NOT OUR OWN.

This observation is at the heart of two vary different notions of God. One a product of the mind of Saint Anselm: the ontological proof of God. God is only one thing, perfect in His completeness. He can "be" no other way than perfect. The second is an historical observation: the great success of Islam. In Islam God is the creator of all things. He is perfect in every attribute. This is the central dogma of Islam. No religion connects its dogmatic and moral theology as intimately as Islam. Anselm pushes man to believe; Islam states a normative certainty.

René Descartes has taken the blame which really should be divided among many for this "divided self" error. He got stuck with the blame for an error that goes back to Plato. The fact is that there is no mind/body problem. The soul exists within the body which has a fragile will to believe (soul). The mind is external to the body as are behavior and demographic data. The central problem is that we don't know what to believe in. There are many parties who seek the use of our "will to believe". Eric Hoffer (*The True Believer*) explains the process of belief better than anyone else. The slender volume which appeared at the beginning of the 1950's explains the past, the present, and the future of the fanatic's behavior.

Words – what do they mean? What are they? Do they represent solely material things? Can they represent abstract concepts? The answer is simple. Language is an imposition of the mind on the brain. One's society imposes on the child a particular language. The brain has the capacity to accept this and build upon it, producing a unique use of the first acquired language(s). I believe that in this particular matter (and virtual no other) Chomsky is nearly correct. He summarizes his view in a highly critical review of Skinner's *Verbal Behavior*. Chomsky states: the scientific application of behavioral principles from animal research is severely lacking in explanatory adequacy and is furthermore, particularly superficial as an account of human verbal behavior because a theory restricting itself to external conditions, to "what is learned", cannot adequately account for the rapid language acquisition of children, including their quickly developing ability to form grammatical sentences, and the universally creative language use of competent native speakers to highlight the ways in which Skinner's view was quite different from that which is observed. He argued that to understand human verbal behavior such as the creative aspects of language use and language development, one must first postulate a genetic linguistic endowment. Here I depart from Chomsky. This capacity is not normative; it takes what it finds outside itself. Abstract concepts may or may not exist. To complete this thought I present two examples. Two people never make love; they just have sex because love does not exist. A soldier doesn't fight in a good war because good doesn't exist within any war. He is simply a killer. Words such as love and courage are errors

Whose echoes live in memory yet,
Though envious years would say "forget."
Lewis Carroll from the opening verses of *Through the Looking Glass*

Here enters Gilbert Ryle whose *The Concept of the Mind* is the great product of logical positivism. Ryle calls these errors (that Hume first recognized) "ghosts in the machine." The mind is external to the body. It is the chief ghost (or error of philosophy) to put the mind within the body. Physicians treat brains. Notions of the reality of abstractions are, according to Ryle, "category errors". Experience (history) denies these words.

I am in Ryle's camp, yet I also champion the "modified realism" of the cosmos with the synthesis of Fitche and Jung (the positive archetypes and normative paradigms). This allows the existence of intangibles which are excluded from Ryle's system.

There is talk of selfish genes, altruistic loci, and sequences of DNA that make us social animals. I suppose that there are people who have time machines hidden in their labs. Such notions are the property of theology. No one can say how primitive humanoids acted. The social aspects of early humanoid existence are veiled and hidden forever. One does not read human history in the genetic code. So far, all we see is various pathologies, and these we often see with myopia.

There are all sorts of behavioral studies and demonstrations that our species is by nature vile. Spinoza could have written our species' epitaph. Let me expand his words. These are the words he read within the human soul: What is good is rare. What is good we refuse to acknowledge. Our evil grinds our souls into powder which the wind blows into every direction of the compass.

Each person has the same desires with slight variation within each desire. One of these is a peculiar desire. This passion is belief itself; William James called this "The will to believe". James meant belief in God. However, this healthy "will" has a great "negative capacity". This use of the term was developed by John Keats; the poet absorbs and is shaped by sensory experience. The soul sucks in whatever is outside. "Garbage in, garbage out": that's the unified field theory of the soul. Be careful of these early statements; they are written on the soul with indelible ink. The soul accepts ambiguity readily. Unlike the complex, sturdy language "hardware", the soul is initially rudimentary and fragile. Strong and complex intellects embedded within souls are uncommon.

CHRIST AND RAPHAEL

Let us now turn to medicine's two of the four great defects which are intertwined one with the other. Medicine is seen as a positive materialistic enterprise; at present, it is such (Defect 1). Our task is to suggest modified realism as a more useful philosophical basis, providing a better theoretical basis for etiology of disease, a greater chance of palliation, and clearer normative guidance. Medicine is too narrow (Defect 2). There is ample space for empiric materialism, modified realism, and a distinct normative orientation (derived from paradigms) within the craft of medicine.

The archangel Raphael represents the ancient archetype of healing (see appendix V). He is the healer. When God cast man out of Eden, *Rophe* became a helper, a servant whose task was to preserve man's mortal life and to treat his diseases. It must be remembered that he alone of all the archangels may work against the will of God. His mission is to preserve mortal life. He is not primarily the servant of God; the Lord has commanded him to serve human life. Recall the Hebrew word for a doctor of medicine is *Rophe* connected to the same root as Raphael.

The name of the archangel Raphael appears only in the Deuterocanonical Book of Tobit. The Book of Tobit is considered canonical by Roman Catholic, Orthodox and some Protestant Christians. Raphael first appears disguised in human form as the travelling companion of the younger Tobias. During the adventurous course of the journey the archangel's protective influence (as a physician protects his patient) is demonstrated especially in the binding of the demon in the desert of Upper Egypt (a reference to neurological illnesses). After the return and the healing of the blindness of the elder Tobias, Azarias makes himself known as "the angel Raphael, one of the seven, who stand before the Lord".

Regarding the healing powers attributed to Raphael, we have little more than his declaration to Tobit (*Tobit*, 12) that he was sent by the Lord to heal him of his blindness) and to deliver Sarah, his daughter-in-law, from Asmodeus the murderer (preserving life).

Among Catholics, he is the patron saint of medical workers. Raphael is sometimes shown (usually on medallions) as standing atop a large fish or holding a caught fish at the end of a line. The angel used a fish's gallbladder to heal Tobit's eyes, and its heart and liver to drive away Asmodeus (the use of natural extracts as medicines).

Christ is not a doctor of medicine, or a general fated to lead a rebellion, nor a deity passing through the world to show off His powers. He has nothing to do with the medical archetypes presented elsewhere in this book. Here we must begin with the three Magi and their gifts. There is gold for King. A priest uses frankincense and myrrh is for the burial of the dead. The Lord of the Universe will be the Priest and

Sacrifice for all of mankind (*Mt 2:11-12*). Matthew continues; in chapter *8:10-13* Jesus does something that no physician would ever do. He orders the healing of someone He has never seen. He shows the authority to go beyond the labor of the physician. In Matthew *9:1-8*, Jesus points out that He is able to forgive sins as well as heal. Is this something no physician could do? The Christ asks which is easier. He is taunting and warning both his friends and his enemies that the afflicted require both. This is a subtle refutation of the Cartesian man. This is a challenge. He asks: who will take the responsibility for individual humans? If the priests fail, and the doctor succeeds, who is to blame? This is Defect 3: the Cartesian man is a convenient excuse for failure. If the priest, the politician, the mystic, etc. fails the patient, is the physician at fault if he succeeds? Doctors are in the healing profession. Here Christ is a philosopher. As with Wittgenstein, Christ asks not for the label, definition, name, or title, the Rabbi demands the use. The word is made "action" just as the Word is made flesh.

In the same chapter *(8:18-26)* He does two things that no physician would ever claim to do: 1) A woman is healed of a chronic hemorrhage by touching His clothing; 2) Jesus mocks death. He says this girl is just sleeping. He takes her hand and the girl awakes. He continues this behavior throughout all the gospels. Jesus feeds five thousands people (*Mark 6:34-44*), reminding people that Moses fed the children of Israel in the desert. Just before He overturns the market in the temple, He curses a fig tree (*Mark 11:12-25*) which symbolizes the barren ground of the unbelievers. Over and over (*Mark 10:46-52, Matthew 17:16-20, Mark 5:30-34*), Jesus makes the person's faith the central issue of the healing. Christ demands faith first. The physician or the Good Samaritan makes no distinction among persons.

Finally, *John 9:1-41*, the Son of Man uses a complex literary metaphor in which He implies that those who don't believe in Him are blind. In the third verse He is very ironic; He sneers at His critics and says a certain man was born blind so Jesus could give him sight. What He really means is that this man who cannot see will see more than any other person that day. All that He does emphasizes the transcendent nature of God. He proclaims that those that eat His bread, unlike the Israelites in Sinai, shall need no further nourishment *(John 6:24-40)*. Those who consume the Eucharist will have no need for physicians because their lives shall be everlasting and healthy. These are the words of Divinity; no honest physician could make such claims. Christ brings victory over death; the doctor struggles against disease and death with no promise of even transient success. This brings to defect 4; we are too haughty. Physicians do not perform miracles. Our success against disease is far less than we pretend. We are less honest than we should be. Moreover, we need to remember self-deception is perilous.

To close, we need to summarize the four fundamental errors.

1. *Doctors are not God, do not carry out God's will, have not a clue what God has planned for anybody.*
2. *Modified realism is better paradigm for medicine than materialism. We are forced to admit to the possibility that there are things beyond the material, outside the rational, and removed from morality: archetypes. Other immaterial "things" which are rational and moral, we shall call paradigms. Paradigms are less common than archetypes, and there are only a limited number of archetypes (perhaps twenty). Marriage and the family are*

a single paradigm. Love isn't; it is not rational and may not be moral. Coitus is a measurable event and is "material". It has a time, place, and a variety of techniques.

3. *People need to be healed; sins need to be forgiven. Somebody has to perform these tasks. It does not matter who does it; it matters that these tasks are done. These two tasks are intertwined because there is no Cartesian man to be divided among various types of shamans.*

4. *Medicine has not been "the science of miracles" that we pretend it to be.*

We have a long way to go before we eradicate these four errors.

THE INDIVISIBLE MAN

Tarry a little: there is something else.
This bond doth give thee here no jot of blood;
The words expressly are 'a pound of flesh:'
Then take thy bond, take thou thy pound of flesh;
But, in the cutting it, if thou dost shed
One drop of Christian blood, thy lands and goods
Are, by the laws of Venice, confiscate
Unto the state of Venice.
*Portia disguised as a doctor of law: Shakespeare's
The Merchant of Venice (1596-1598) Act IV, Scene 1*

The body, the brain, and the soul are united within the individual. Demographic data, the mind, and behavior are external to the individual and are to varying degrees products of the individual and his environment. If you do not believe in God, then the existence of the soul is irrelevant. If you do believe in God, then at death the soul leaves the body and the mind for individual salvation, collective union, abolition of self, or some other fate. Opinions concerning the body may be divided into a spectrum. There is an axis of materialism. The body exists as a material object at one end. At the other end of the axis, life is a dream so all is an illusion including our physical presence. Since this is a book about medicine, we will discard the concept of phantoms diagnosing and treating ghosts. Medicine assumes that the body and its contents are real. It further assumes that physicians are real material objects/persons whose activities affect other material objects/persons.

The body may be a coffin for the soul. Saint Augustine and Saint Bernard thought of the body as a coffin containing rotting, sinful flesh, corrupting the soul. Thus, Saint Bernard's injunction against the study of medicine makes perfect sense. Again since this book is about medicine and since medicine is supposed to be a practical enterprise, we discard these opinions emanating from these two great saints. (These guys are not the people you want attending to you in the emergency room. If you are as Saint Bernard said "a combination of feces and maggots" [my translation from his Latin], he would not do much to save your life.) It must be admitted that the behavior of these two is discordant. Augustine's indulgence of the flesh is well-known. Bernard is a more difficult case. From the modern perspective, he was the enemy of philosophy and the promoter of the Second Crusade. He also was a "miraculous" healer. He despised the study of medicine, but he seems to have gotten the job done. Moreover, he halted numerous episodes of "ethnic cleansing."

Saint Benedict encouraged the study of medicine as well as every other practical craft. He had a more reasonable attitude. Saint Thomas Aquinas took the view that the body was the instrument by which God enlightened man. Certainly, these ideas are more congenial to medicine. The theoretical aim of medicine is to cure. As one of my professors used to remind me, "the patient comes not for diagnosis, but for treatment".

Don't let the author surprise the reader too much, but Batman, Superman, and all the rest don't exist. There are a very few women who are nuns during the day and strippers at night. Moreover, unfortunately for many sadomasochistic young girls, I never have run into any vampires sleeping in coffins. And I have seen a lot of coffins. Alfred Adler put it perfectly. *We are not divisible into two symmetrical or antagonistic selves.* Even Carl Jung does not permit the opposing factor (e.g., male, female; extrovert, introvert; old sage, innocent infant; etc.) to dominate the individual. To Jung the male is heterosexual, or he is abnormal, suffering from a pathological imbalance. There is the dominant and the submissive figure which coincides with genetic sex. Certainly, one may be critical of Jung; however, his point is that we not divisible into a plethora of his quaint figures. The child, the wise old man, the female figure of the muse, the masculine achiever, etc. do not function normally if they are not placed in their "proper places" to form a unique and integrated individual. One may be tempted to call this arrangement the glass menagerie of the individual: unique and easily destroyed. Health is the integration of these pieces into a unified entity.

Thus, the skeptical author of this book believes only under very specific circumstances that bread and wine are the flesh of a God become man. Thus, the meek male dresses as Zorro for the carnival. It is just a game. There are no double lives. There are people who are psychotic, people who are in fugue states, and people who are just plain liars. A person is a singular, unique creature who may pretend to be, but is not someone else. He is most often venal and petty, full of ignorance and false pride. To put it more politely, a psychologist would say such a person has many defense mechanisms.

I got some more bad news: there are no little green men with great big heads riding around in tall spaceship shooting death rays. In the words of Walt Kelly's comic page character, Pogo, "We have met the enemy, and he is us" (from the *Pogo Papers, 1953)*. The only invaders on this planet shooting lethal missiles are members of own species. The psychological term is projection.

The reader will demand to know how I can be so sure that that the body and soul are not distinct. The answer comes from my personal experience. The induction of hypoglycemia by exogenous insulin induces stress responses. Anxiety occurs if the experimenter does not explain that emotional disturbance is an effect of the hormone. If one injects insulin in high enough doses without the knowledge of the subject, the subject will experience anxiety before convulsions and perhaps coma. The same is true of epinephrine. Instead of coma, the heart just wears itself out. Psycho-physiological stress is real. One cannot isolate emotion from the physiology of the body. The body may be a "machine" (Descartes uses the term); however, it is highly complex and unified device. Moreover, I have not seen a human reproduced by other mechanism than a zygote. It is hardly in the same class as the steam engine. Here we connect feeling with physiology. The classical property of emotion is linked to a pharmacological intrusion.

The neurotoxicity of drugs is the proof of this connection. The malfunction of the thyroid is another example. Insufficient secretion of the thyroid hormones classically leads to depression which responds to replacement of the hormone. Anti-depressants are generally not very effective. In contrast, agents that relax the patient such as anti-anxiety agents are more effective in cases of excessive thyroid function. However, these medications are temporary measures. Surgery, "anti-thyroid drugs" and/or radioactive iodine are considered definitive therapies. Brain and body are linked.

Excuse me for being repetitive, but the argument for the indivisibility of the soul in the living human is even more obvious. The soul is present at conception; however, it is extremely fragile. There are two things that will injure or destroy the soul during life. The first is an error in the target of the "will to believe". Much like the monkey exposed to the robot mother or the goose who "believes" that the bearded fellow with a bucket of food is his mother, the soul can be deceived. The proper goal for the soul is to serve God. This may take many forms. The policeman, the fireman, the scientist, the priest, the physician: all may live in the service of God, if their intentions are to do good or to discover truth. There is no other proper target for the soul. In my opinion, atheism or any other *ism* besides Theism is wrong. Of course, if there is no God, there is still within each the "will to believe in something. So, if the intentions are good at the beginning, what can destroy them? A grave illness or injury can prevent the soul's development; this is not the fault of the individual. An addiction to narcotics or stimulants destroys the will. Thus, there is no will to believe in anything except the next dose. (I will not discuss the various reasons for illicit use) Nevertheless, one cannot overlook the most prominent reason for the soul's failure to mature. There is a list of tasks outlined by Erik Erikson; there are "seven labors" before the soul is mature. You can't skip any. There is Maslow's pyramid. You can't get to spiritual fulfillment without climbing all the steps of this structure. The conclusion is clear, the task of the Church is to get the individual to accomplish the first seven labors and/or climb the pyramid. Either one is sufficient because they are different ways to express the same social/biological tasks. So, you got to have the right target, and there is only one way to hit that target. As Kermit the frog put it: "It aint easy being green." Failure is common. The products of such failures are described by Eric Hoffer in his slim catalogue of human weakness and mendacity. The reader will not be surprised that Hoffer cannot resist assigning blame to religion (especially the Roman Catholic Church, Islam, and his favorite target, St. Paul) itself as well as the society in both the individual and the Church exist. The infant is born which depending on your beliefs is either a positive fact or a normative good.   Remember the rule: bad may come from good, but good cannot emerge from bad.   There is another side to this argument concerning the soul. The theological argument has been mentioned previously.

Well, as I was saying, there was a man called Cardinal Newman...Meanwhile, listen to what this old Arch-Community-Songster said..."We are not our own any more than what we possess is our own. We did not make ourselves; we cannot be supreme over ourselves... We are God's property..."
(Aldous Huxley, *Brave New World*, Chapter Seventeen)

That's the mission of the physician: to save God's creature upon whom He has showered grace which the human race has spurned in favor of rebellion based upon arrogance and ignorance. Sure, you can say there is no God. But there is plenty of smallpox virus being stockpiled. There are many nations with nuclear weapons. Not only is the evilness of man a problem for the theologian, this is a problem for evolutionists: we have evolved into the species that will extinguish itself. For those who believe in special creation, they must admit God did a fairly lousy job. However, these are not the physician's problems.

Perhaps, the physician can help his patient survive long enough to complete the long and treacherous path to the Temple. Maslow's spiritual plane is high. Maslow's requirements are too rigorous. Not everybody can climb Everest or K2 without oxygen or a guide. Erikson's criteria are sufficiently demanding. His pyramid is high enough. There are no gondolas, no hot air balloons, and no helicopters. You climb alone for the most part before reaching the Temple.

True are the words of Euclid to one of the Hellenistic pharaoh: "there is no road to understanding geometry. The great human master of geometry; Spinoza, will tell you that which is good is rare. Wittgenstein's last notebooks speak to the damaged receptor, the vessel that we call the soul. The great saint of logical positivism died with "unreasonable hope" (faith) in God whom he could never delineate. We, physicians, have no such problem; we have the archetypes.

THIS SIDE OF PARADISE

Physicians began as priests in Egypt, in the Fertile Crescent (Modern Iraq), Anatolia (part of Modern Turkey), and Greece. Between 1200 BC and 300 BC, the temple and the physician parted ways in all these places. The physician became the enemy of the priest.

In our little pageant of heaven and hell, we have described the seven angels. Of these two are indifferent to the physician. Michael and Gabriel have their own separate tasks. The virtues of physician are far different from that of another type of man. As we will see he must be a type of priest without divine power and with the greatest discretion in his conduct. The physician's enemies are Satan (pride), Beelzebub (ignorance), and human frailty as well as indiscretion (gluttony, promiscuity, use of illicit substances). So, who helps the doctor? There is always Mephistopheles with his ideas; however, the physician must adapt these tips to the situation. Most of all there is Raphael whose task is the healing of mankind, both individual humans and the species as a whole. But there is this tension between God and the physician. Remember the son of Apollo, Aesculapius. His father Apollo killed his mother because she was unfaithful. Zeus killed the first physician because he was interfering with the natural order of things. Not enough people were dying to satisfy Hades. Maybe, Aesculapius took money for his work. Zeus took offence to the fact that poor

Aesculapius had to support his family. The idea that the son of a lesser deity needed income did not matter to Zeus. But after the murder of their patron, his priests lived in palaces called temples, were rich, and always had their bellies full. It could be that Zeus ran out of thunderbolts or that the patients ran out of patience with Zeus. In the "deity business", the god does not have to be dead. Being unemployed (*under implored*) is equally fatal. This is a problem that Dionysus and Demeter never had: Who doesn't want a glass of wine and a sandwich? You need bread and wine. Christ knew which "material objects" to use.

Christianity began as a non-political faith. But it divided itself into three *modus operandi*: first there was the non-political faith which managed to contain all the knowledge necessary for human existence. The Italian Benedictines managed to have huge libraries, full of practical information. The civilization was dependent on this knowledge. No other institution had such knowledge. The same was true in Ireland and England. The second type of Christianity began as the first but developed into a strange creature. The same faith became part of new nations. There was the Greek Orthodox, Russian Orthodox, Georgian Orthodox, Rumanian Orthodox, etc. The third type of Christianity is quite similar to Islam. The words of Luther and John Calvin were heard because the political units in which they were heard had grown weary of some Roman commanding them.

There's the problem with religion. A successful religion must be the fountain of all practical knowledge. The faith born on Mt. Sinai and nurtured by thousands of pages of scripture could not afford to fail. It did not because it held special knowledge. Its members would tolerate endless persecution. The same is true of Zoroaster's followers in Iran (where they still suffer severe repression) and in India where they have thrived. Islam failed. At present, it mocks the West while Islamic states long for technological and financial equality with the West. They seem to have adopted Janus as their second deity. (Northern Europe during the medieval centuries had no such aspirations. In fact, St. Bernard found too many Jewish and Muslim ideas in Aquinas' work). The Protestants especially in North America surrendered to secular forces. The Catholic Church became the enemy of certain categories of scholarship. So, what happened?

The reader must realize that the venerable Hippocrates broke totally with religion. He was essentially a student of Aristotle. He thought God to be irrelevant to his profession. He did not deny God; he simply demanded that his followers live in a way that was honorable to the profession. As medicine progressed, there was an obvious conflict between religion that sees that life begins with death and the honorable physician whose vow is to preserve life. This was even of the less worthy medics who were more astrologers than doctors Chaucer describes these fellows best: "His studies was but little on the Bible" (line 440 of *The General Prologue* of *The Canterbury Tales*) But temple and dispensary have a new argument. Today Christianity champions certain physicians over others because it has embraced "the dignity of the individual human life". This regard arose from two factors:

1) People began finding less pleasure in the Spanish Inquisition as spectators. What's

more, hanging witches put a big dent in the work week.

2) About two hundred years ago, medicine became effective in alleviating suffering (narcotics). Seventy years ago medicine became effective in therapeutics.

There is a profound problem in medicine that will be the subject of a later chapter. This problem may be state very simply: the knowledge of the physician should not be used to kill or injure others. The business of the physician is not to do God's will, not to serve the state as an executioner, not to make life for more convenient for one person by murdering another as an abortionist. The reader is now perfectly aware that the author is in a tiny minority, a pariah to the amoral commerce of modern medical practice in which the patient is either a source of income or the grudging liability of a socialist state. The reader will also realize that it is indeed irrelevant where the physician is a theist or atheist, classic Greek or contemporary American. The physician's ideology is simple: preserve man's life. Like the Good Samaritan (*Luke, 10:30-37)* the doctor serves the individual. The greatest exhortation to rational and civil behavior flows from the lips of Moses *(Deuteronomy 30:11-20)*. He speaks of God, but observes that civility and prosperity are necessary in a healthy, thriving nation (*Deuteronomy: 31, 32, and 33)*.

The physician is not to use his patients as experimental subjects without very good reason (i.e., the benefit to the patient is the only goal for the experiment). Human knowledge should not be based on the placing persons in the same normative category as laboratory rats or microbes. Finally, and this is painful to say, the physician does not know God's will nor should he care about It; the doctor's business is preserving life, improving what cannot be cured, and maintaining the dignity of the person. Just like Raphael in the book of Tobit, the physician is sent by God to assist humanity.

SCIENTIFIC MEDICINE

From 1500 on, there were at most only three sciences First there was physics. Then from physics and alchemy came chemistry. Biology sprung from "natural philosophy" and the proof that the laws of physics and the very few rules of chemistry applied equally to living and non-living things.

Some would stay that all science is physics. Mathematics is how science expresses itself after it has gone beyond simple description (which is a very difficult thing). It's hard to be objective in your description, and it's even harder to induce from specific examples general rules. Science is an inductive process. It goes from the specific to the general. Conversely, deduction applies the rules derived from induction to produce a specific conclusion about a particular case. For example, you purchase a book which describes all the ducks found on the coast of Virginia. You have purchased someone's descriptions and the inductions derived from these specific observations. Now you may make deductions based on previous inductive reasoning.

Medicine must not go from theory to practice; it must go from experience to standards of practice. It cannot invoke spirits; it must deal with the flesh and the world. Finally, the history of medicine is a complex and controversial subject clouded by cultural and social biases. The beginning of the Renaissance was the rediscovery of the Greek language; it may have been the Attic Greek of Athens' Golden Age, the Ionic prose of the Hippocratic corpus, the *Koine* of the New Testament, or the polished cosmopolitan Greek of Galen. Michelangelo studied anatomy for art's sake. Leonardo drew man from the uterus of the floating fetus to the deathbed of old age in his secret notebooks. It was the dissectors who overthrew the old ways of seeing man. Later, the microscope and the surgeon's knife would reveal much more.

There are two ways to do anything. One is scientific; the other is not. The scientific method is confined to a particular form of investigation. Science is positive: it makes no claim about the moral value of its findings. It begins with an open mind, and it continues in its comparison between a control and an experimental group. Or it may begin with any hypothesis which it seeks to prove or disprove. It is easier to present examples of what is not scientific. For example, one goes out to some Pacific Island and describes the behavior of its native tribes. It could be an interesting book, but it's not science. However, if the observer divided the tribe into those who were cannibals and those who were not, then the observer noted that the cannibals demonstrated neurological symptoms and had abnormal brains at autopsy. Additionally those that were never cannibals had no such lesion at post-mortem examination. That is science. That's Nobel Prize material. This example is a central part of that tiny fraction of medicine that is truly scientific. Conversely, if one knows the identity of a suspect and runs a DNA test seeking that suspect solely, one rejects science. The concept of knowing what you are supposed to find nullifies any notion of objectivity. Forensic samples should be run without the police providing a list of names. To be blunt, the person who collects the sample and the person who analyzes it should be different.

Science is not concern with guilt or innocence. Neither is science interested in good or bad, nor in successful or unsuccessful therapies. When the physician goes from the laboratory to the bed side, he most often changes from scientist into one of two characters: the rational thinker or the witch doctor. He is a healer (or at least he should be). For the purpose of medicine is to cure, to treat, to palliate. None of these are scientific. The shaman acts as a magician. This is not always the case. The rational physician acts upon a number of propositions which are expanded by "formal logic". In reality rational physicians are in the minority, and even they often act as shamans

Science accepts the notion of cause-and-effect. Though daily life would difficult to bear without this concept, science is impossible without this paradigm. Science accepts the validity of causality as something that may exist within the mind and surely exists outside of it. This is the opposite of what many philosophers believe to be correct. Moreover, the use of the term causality here is simple: an event occurs as a result of prior event: no chains of events, everything -- one step at a time, every step isolated from the next and from the previous.

Science is about measuring things. It begins in the material world. And we must recall that not everything that is real can be measured at a particular juncture in time. Now we can see viruses and photograph the shadows of molecules. These things were always there; we simply could not record their presence in the past. To confirm a hypothesis is to test the utility of a specific explanation. To perceive, to measure, and to calibrate are attempts to deal in causality: there is a linkage between the thermometer and fever, between radar and airplanes. This association is termed cause-and-effect because it is reassuring to do so. Causality is a house of cards. Such associations should usually be termed called correlations. Provable causality is uncommon

To clarify this, let us take the example of a person throwing a switch to turn on a lamp. It cannot be said with absolute certainty that there is a causal relationship between the switch and the lamp. Leibniz would tell us that the monads are in harmony. Malebranche would say God knows the fellow wanted illumination and made it happen. One could spend a life time defending these "strange" theories. Instead, allow Hume to assure us that these two events cannot be shown to be linked by causality. One may say that the throwing of the switch and the bulb supplying light are highly correlated; their chance of being independent events is very small. No one thinks there is a little man inside the lamp who sees somebody flick a switch and then if he feels up to it starts to glow. However, the relationship of the glowing bulb and the person who perceives the light is quite different. The person says: "I see something that I have learned to call light. The cause is the sensing of a particular category of event; the effect is the naming of the phenomenon. It is internal to the brain and a matter of linguistics for the mind.

CHANCE AND CIRCUMSTANCE

1865: Mendel read his paper, "Experiments on Plant Hybridization", at the Natural History Society of Brünn in Moravia in 1865. When Mendel's paper was published in 1866 in "Proceedings of the Natural History Society of Brünn", it had little impact. It is the single most significant document in the history of biology. Mendel destroyed "special creation" and determinism, replacing them with the roll of a die. Nevertheless...

Laroche himself is a student of orchids, and he narrates a poetic passage about the limitless shapes that orchids can take in attracting insects ... There is even one orchid so strangely shaped that Darwin hypothesized a moth with a 12-inch proboscis that

could dip down into its long, hollow tube. Such a
moth was actually found.
From Roger Ebert's essay on the "Great Movie"
Adaptation (based on *The Orchid Thief*, by Susan
Orlean which was based on the life of John Laroche.
(I stole this from Ebert's essay of 18 September,
2008. Some steal orchids; I steal …)

Ebert also wrote that neither the insect nor the flower
had the least idea that such adaptation was occurring.
He says neither component realizes what itself nor its
compliment is doing. This is not surprising. The easy
answer is that God does the thinking for them. The
human inclination is that such perfect fits between
couples are long in the planning. However, in my
experience, I never found that insects or flowers are
long range planners. They seem not to have any
capacity for cogitation. So, they realize nothing; they
do not know the history of their species. One can
read many speculative volumes about how this

particular moth and orchid got together. There were others who tried figured out why Mr. Laroche got so enthusiastic about orchids. I do not think that everything has a reason to explain it. The orchid and the moth form such a relationship: there is absence of causality. Mr. Laroche merits analysis. But which one? The actual person, the character in the novel, the character in the film, the actor playing the character, and the screenwriter are all candidates. Which one is the real Laroche? It is that pesky mind/brain/soul/body problem. Does the novelist understand more about Laroche than Laroche himself? Is the screenwriter in an analogous position to the novelist in a parallel universe? Personally, I'd just grab Laroche and try to get rid of all the Hollywood nonsense. If I could do that, I could begin an analysis of the individual. But first I would have to find him. We've been able to conjure up at least five "Laroches". And, if I found *him*, I would have to study his behavior because, as Gilbert Ryle tells us, we cannot read people's thoughts (even if they are spoken or written: people lie, make mistakes, and misuse language). All this should put some points in Mr. Hume's column. Discarding the Cartesian man makes medicine tougher. Take a careful history and analyze it carefully. Of course, this is not efficient. It takes time. It is bad business, costs too much money to take the time. The only argument in favor of this meta-linguistic, non-Cartesian analysis is that it produces more right diagnoses. Of course, not every patient needs such analysis.

This is neither evolution nor progress; the objective is surviving for another reproductive cycle. Existence is a positive attribute; there is no normative aspect here. Sad to say the loyal canine, the resourceful monkey, and the other "characters" Darwin fills his books with are projections (category errors). Alligators and sharks kill because they are predators (positive statement). Lions most often kill for food. Darwin writes that he deplores slavery constantly; he must have realized that natural selection has nothing to with which man is chained and which holds the key.

We need to return to Christ's biography for a single incidence in which He poses a very practical question concerning the profession of medicine. This is repetition.

23: Whether is easier, to say, Thy sins be forgiven thee; or to say, Rise up and walk?
24: But that ye may know that the Son of man hath power upon earth to forgive sins, (he said unto the sick of the palsy,) I say unto thee, Arise, and take up thy couch, and go into thine house.
25: And immediately he rose up before them, and took up that whereon he lay, and departed to his own house, glorifying God.

There are many folks lying immobile on their cots. Who is going to make them walk? We repeat: the patient did not come to hear a lecture; he came to be cured. Any rational patient would have a greater interest in the therapy than the therapist.

THE CANCER WITHIN

I was struck with a profound veneration at the sight of Brutus, and could easily discover the most consummate virtue, the greatest intrepidity and firmness of mind, the truest love of his country, and general benevolence for mankind, in every lineament of his countenance. I observed, with much pleasure, that these two persons were in good intelligence with each other; and Caesar freely confessed to me, "that the greatest actions of his own life were not equal, by many degrees, to the glory of taking it away."
J. Swift, *Gulliver's Travels* Book 3, Chapter 7

From Gulliver's rough draft of 1722, published in two installments in 1726.

... It could be said that the first period – 1500-1660 – was dominated by the issue of what to believe in religion; the second – 1661-1789 – by what to do about the status of the individual ...; the third – 1790-1920 – by what means the individual achieve social and economic equality.
Jacques Barzun, *From Dawn to Decadence*, page XXI

Barzun misunderstands a fundamental social change (op. cit., pp 688-89). Barzun talks about Liberalism's "Great Switch" to Socialism. This never occurred in Germany or the United States during the first decades of the last century. They were prevented by particular politicians of the nineteenth century. From Hamilton to Bismarck, Nationalism used Liberalism as a defense for increasing the power of the state. Friedman (*Free to Choose*, 1979) spends several passages of *Free to Choose* criticizing Alexander

Hamilton. He points out Hamilton's protection of American industry on page 27. From page 40 through 42, Hamilton is the enemy of free trade.

The control of the national economy was to rest in a National Bank; this is a notion that Friedman despised. Andrew Jackson managed to abolish such institution. Woodrow Wilson (the secretive mandarin of the presidency) rammed the Federal Reserve System through the Congress, pretending it to be a benefit of a big hearted government, fighting for the "little man". It was nothing of the kind. Similarly, Lincoln waved The Manifesto of Secession (the Declaration of Independence) to justify four bloody years of war to prevent a secession that would have fragmented the United States. Instead of a world power, if Lincoln had failed, two or more nations would have played the game of European powers: Alliance and Betrayal.

Bismarck never had any interest in socialism (again contrary to Friedman's statement op. cit. page. 90). He was interested in a reliable and healthy workforce. He was building a nation, not handing out alms to the poor. That's why the German, system has worked so well in contrast to the Beaverbrook model of Britain or the welfare state model of the United States. The emphasis was on producing a workforce in every field of endeavor. In the process, poverty was slowly and incompletely defeated. It was not all inconclusive or perfect.

But it was better than the situation that currently exists in the United States because Bismarck had coupled productivity with health. The entire premise of a political or social "right to healthcare" is an absurd concept. There are two other justifications for *the* "right to health care". One is theological; the other is scientific. We shall address them later.

Hamilton, Lincoln, Bismarck, and Wilson cared nothing for the poor; they were interested in national power. Barzun's great switch was an illusion in Germany and a reality in Britain. This explains how a single nation destroyed the greatest empire the world has ever known. Even the stupidity of the Nazis could not completely undermine Bismarck's achievements. The United States between Lincoln and Wilson, despite weak presidents with the exception of G. Cleveland and T. Roosevelt, was by 1917 *the world power*. Currently Russia, China, a coalition of Islamic states, and India challenge the United States and so far none has displaced it. But the future is guaranteed to no man, tribe, or nation. In 1914 the British sterling was the standard; by 1918 it was the Yankee dollar was the reference for international trade.

Efficient nationalized medicine is a unitary system for working citizens, soldiers, children, with careful monitoring of maternity and child-rearing behavior among the parents and the welfare of those retired or disabled from private or public service. With rare exceptions, co-payments should modest but omnipresent. Except for research and academic purposes, there should no provision for free care.

The cancer within is the notion of a political right to health care. It is the "bread and circuses" attitude of the bloated empire. Something for nothing, satisfying the incredible *appétit* of the mob, running to patients who would be better served by a simple set of instructions, and many acts of folly are the daily bread of socialist medicine. Low quality medical care available to all is no real benefit.

The notion of a political right to medical care is absurd. There is no right to housing or food. We have only those rights which we, as individuals, can defend and/or earn. This is why the citizen votes and pays taxes. God has endowed us with liberty; the Lexus is up to us.

The cancer is too much government. The government should exist to establish a level playing field (regulation is analogous to the baseball umpire), provide economic stability. The purpose of the military is to maintain stable economic conditions and safe trade. Education is critical to the future. A stable and solvent pensioned class provides a guarantee and motivation to the workers. Government hires teachers for the young and policemen to protect all. The protection of the individual, property rights, and the economy should be the goal of government. Education tops the list of government imperatives.

For those nations without such a system, failure is likely. There is no point in using gentle words. As with the Japanese of 170 years ago, such change is to be coerced. Japan had to modernize or be destroyed. China was a paper dragon before the brutality of Japanese conquest (Friedman, op. cit. pp. 137-8). The Middle Kingdom has yet to learn the "rules of the game". China and Russia chose suicidal civil wars. India is now four separate nations. Three of these are at war internally and externally. The fourth

(Bangladesh) cannot afford to be at war with itself or anybody else. It remains inept in its economic policy. A different defect holds back Islam; religion is a private matter, rarely discussed during economic transactions. Keep your social peculiarities well hidden. The game played by world power has rules and a dress code.

IGNORANCE, SLOTH, AND DESIRE

Adam Smith published *The Wealth of Nations* in 1776. There were few efficacious medicines. Birth was a duel between life and death for both mother and child. Surgery was in the hands of barbers in Britain and academics in Italy. Medical practice in Adam Smith's world differed vastly from our time.

However, the same institutions still interact in every field of human endeavor, and they are most often competitors. There are still margins of profit. In the grocery business, these margins are thin. Yet, there are plenty of places to buy food in developed countries. The concept of absolute value exists. Diamonds are "a girl's best friend". However, in the desert a bucket of water has a higher absolute value.

Health has a lowest absolute value for many until they get sick. The profit margin of physicians and other providers in the medical field vary widely. This is mostly due to interference by the medical profession, the legal profession, and the government. As I write this the United States and possibly the rest of the world are in the worst economic crisis since the great depression. Moreover, we haven't even eradicated smallpox. Nobody knows how many batches are left; there are suppose to be only two. We have spent all this money and life expectancy is either stable or declining in 2009. Let us not prolong the discussion. Allow me to come straight to the conclusion: we cannot afford to spend vast sums to constantly error in our medical care. We know better; we just don't do better.

Professor Smith would tell us somebody is able to come in and do a better job. We have huge demand, purportedly a vast fund of practical knowledge, and lots of money to spend. So, what happened? In the last chapter we noted a political rationale for universal healthcare. Here we should make the case for the persons not covered by Bismarck's system. We begin with a question. Which institution has the most to gain from covering those not protected? These are the same institutions that will decrease the profit margin because of the competitive nature of its members. Here comes the theological reason for universal health care.

Organized religion is the answer. God is in Heaven; sick people are here on earth. God has redeemed man and justified human dignity. However, His institutional representatives on earth have defended the dignity of each person and the right to live within a compassionate and just social order poorly or not at all. If you can set up a system of competitive conversion based upon the ability to delivery food, shelter, and healthcare, then you have a market. It is in the interest of these entities to tear down the professional, legal, and governmental barriers that are in place. It is only the ignorance and sloth of the various sets that prevents this aggressive form of conversion. Substitute the suicide bomber and the howling preacher with food and healthcare. What is lacking is the desire; what is present is narcissism. So, stop looking at your image in the mirror, and get out your binoculars. Get educated. Remember the depositary of knowledge is also the dwelling of power. Either you as a church want to do good works or you are simply another Ponzi scheme. I am not impressed by pious declarations. Religion should contest the actions of the government; various churches should compete for members by doing the most for their members. Monolithic societies are the greatest enemy of all; the oligarchy (secular and/or religious) benefit only so long as they can hold their positions on the apex of the pyramid. Remember Humpty Dumpty was pushed. To add another nursery school paradigm: there were ten little Indians. At the end, there was only one, and his name was the State (the modern oligarchs). Bismarck's plan is the best for the state; it is not always the best for the individual.

I would be impressed by good food, clean water, community hygiene, and low disease prevalence all the same time for every member of the open community where faiths compete with syringes not rifles. That would be a miracle. You say God's on your side, show me. So far, there is no need to be awed. Instead, I see this…

George Orwell and Aldous Huxley got it just right. The fate of man without God and with single monolithic government is either the loss of liberty with genetic modification of the species, free drugs, unlimited coitus or the loss of liberty with cheap gin, repressive sexual practices, and endless war.

Hobbs reminded us several centuries before that if the individual and the state came into conflict, the individual has a particular freedom, the free will to choose death. This is not scene from the future but a description from the middle of the last century which would have astounded Hobbs.

The voice from the telescreen was still pouring forth its tale of prisoners and booty and slaughter shouting. One of them approached with the gin bottle. Winston, sitting in a blissful dream, paid no attention as his glass was filled up. He was not running or cheering any longer. He was back in the Ministry of Love, with everything forgiven, his soul white as snow. He was in the public dock, confessing everything, implicating everybody. He was walking down the white-tiled corridor, with the feeling of walking in sunlight, and an armed guard at his back. The long hoped-for bullet was entering his brain. ...O stubborn, self-willed exile from the loving breast! But it was all right, everything was all right, the struggle was finished. He had won the victory over himself. He loved Big Brother.

George Orwell, *1984*, 1949, from the last two paragraphs of the novel

Render unto Caesar…These have been the consequences of religion's retreat into the safe walls of its churches, its "fear and trembling" behind closed doors!

Parritt: (speaking of Hickey) Yes, but he isn't the only one who needs peace, Larry… He's lucky. He's through, now… You remember what Mother's like, Larry…As long as she lives, she'll never be able to forget what I've done to her even in her sleep… Jesus, Larry, can't you say something? …
Larry: go! Get the hell out of life … before I choke out it out of you! Go up -!
Act IV, *The Iceman Cometh,* Eugene O'Neill, written in 1939, produced 1946; Fragments from Vintage edition.

This is the culture of death that flowered in the sad summer of 1912 during which Harry Hope and his barflies experienced another season in dystopia. Let's talk about young Parrit. The Goddess of Reason, and the honest skeptic (who was an idealist seduced by the

Goddesses of 1789, 1848, etc.) brought into this unfeeling, indifferent world a son, Parritt. His mother had no love for him. She had the Cause. The authorities wanted the goddess, the anarchist harridan. So her son gave her glorious martyrdom. Larry wanted neither his old ideas nor his young son. Larry did not acknowledge his son; however, the "burnt out case" opened the possibility of suicide for his son. This seems a perversion of another archetype, does it not?

AQUINAS FOR PHYSICIANS

One moment now, Mr. Dedalus, and you will see. There is an art in lighting a fire. We have the liberal arts and we have the useful arts. This is one of the useful arts.

--I will try to learn it, said Stephen.

--Not too much coal, said the dean, working briskly at his task, that is one of the secrets.

James Joyce, *Portrait of the Artist*, 1914-1917, chapter 5

We will shift from the obligations of the state and other institutions to those of the individual physician.

The reader can see (Appendix I) how the author has vivisected Thomas.

Archetypes are positive and make no reference to rational or normative statements. Cardinal Newman's statement is an archetype, perhaps the most profound Western archetypes. Man kills man; man kills God. Man eats God and man. God restores His ownership that was forfeited after the Fall. Before the Fall of Adam and Eve, there was master-client relationship between God and mankind. The relationship between patricians and plebeians of the Roman republic is a pale model of this preternatural relation. The physician and patient have a vastly different connection. The physician is the wise servant to his patient. He is a servant regulated by a particular paradigm.

Paradigms may or may not be rational; they are always normative. Hippocrates or Raphael or

Apollo's son may be loosely thought of as archetypes. Only the third is a true archetype. It is empty of moral consistency. The Hippocratic and the healing angel "archetypes" are completely normative. They are strictly speaking paradigms. Here's the paradigm of the ideal physician.

Wisdom- The gift of wisdom perfects a person's speculative reason in matters of judgment about the truth. Correct.

Knowledge - The gift of knowledge perfects a person's practical reasoning in matters of judgment about the truth. Correct. But the second is achieved before the first: knowledge comes before wisdom

Judgment - The gift of counsel perfects a person's practical reason in the apprehension of truth and allows the person to respond prudently, moved through the research of reason. Correct.

Courage -The gift of courage allows people the firmness of mind.

Understanding - Also called "Common Sense." The gift of understanding perfects a person's speculative reason in the apprehension of truth. It is the gift whereby self-evident principles are known. Incorrect, nothing is self-evident in medicine. Do not trust, verify

Piety - Piety is the gift whereby, we pay worship and duty to God as our Father. Interesting notion! However, as Jacob Marley put it:

"Mankind is my business" Prayers with eyes toward heaven are easy as long as the starving, sad multitude is kept at a distance. I have no need to repeat Huxley's quotation about that old singer Cardinal Newman.

Let us present the second list. In *Summa Theologica* II.2, Thomas Aquinas asserts the following correspondences between the seven Capital Virtues and the seven Gifts of the Holy Spirit.

*The gift of wisdom corresponds to the virtue of charity. This is professionalism for the physician. Not charity, but duty, is the command

*The gift of knowledge corresponds to the virtue of faith. For the doctor, knowledge is a slippery slope whose efficacy is always under scrutiny: dismiss faith, embrace doubt. Think before you act. Jesus would agree; he was a carpenter. Measure twice, cut once.

*The gift of counsel corresponds to the virtue of prudence. Here no modification is needed. It is the greatest of virtue. Reserve what you hear and see; tell no one of the illnesses of your patients. Consider all normative aspects before performing positive acts.

*The gift of fortitude corresponds to the virtue of fortitude. The flesh is weak; the physician is always tested by all the seven deadly sins. Avarice, lust, envy, and the others tug at your coat constantly. Resist them.

*The gift of understanding corresponds to the virtue of faith. Replace the word faith with scrutiny. Your understanding often comes from the death of others. We learn from the dying; we must not ignore such understanding (paid for in the currency of human life) as we treat the living.

*The gift of piety corresponds to the virtue of justice. We are the advocates of our patients and the defenders of life.

*The gift of fear of the Lord corresponds to the virtue of hope. We have not the time to consider abstracts such as God's will which we cannot know or society's interest which may be irrelevant, trivial, or malignant. For example, the avoidance of social embarrassment does not justify the murder of the unborn. Using the "right to life" to justify experimentation that benefits the physician, but turns the person from human to a number in a protocol is disgusting.

Repetition is the mother of study. We will repeat them. What are these divinely imposed positive archetypes and moral paradigms? James Joyce uses linguistic terms which describe the medium and the messages of these "divine" or "universal" intrusions. As always there are layers and layers of meaning in this "simple" complaint:

I cannot speak or write these words without unrest of spirit. His language, so familiar and so foreign, will always be for me an acquired speech. I have not made or accepted its words. My voice holds them at bay. My soul frets in the shadow of his language. *Portrait of the Artist*, 1914-1917, chapter 5

This is how man relates to God. This is how the physician attempts to master his profession. We must master this strange language full of archetypes, paradigms, and category errors. For the believer, God mastered this language to communicate with man. Man is indivisible; there is daylight world which seems (after accepting certain assumptions) is common to all. And there is the night world of sleep and shadows where the only lights are archetypes. This latter world is particular to each person with the archetypes and paradigms in a unique arrangement. No two persons have the same dark world. When Ryle says we cannot see our thoughts or those of others, it is because he disregarded one of the basic tenets of pre-Socratic philosophy. He forgot "the language, so familiar and so foreign". The priests in the old temples did not need God whispering in their ears. They knew "the acquired speech"

Yet the brain carries with it guilt and remorse. It's most often hidden, escaping the brain and entering the mind or the comportment of the individual. Sometimes, it is stuck in the mind (Macbeth's "dagger of the mind"). These "daggers of the mind" often bring their owners to the doctor. They compel the patient to be sick. Some people confess to a cleric and are relieved of the burden. Others rationalize guilt which means culpability appears disguised as peculiar habits. The police often bring these to the physician's attention. Others manage to destroy guilty completely with self-deception and/or pharmacological intervention (licit and illicit)

So, is a requirement that we steal the priest's stole (a badge of authority, a necktie draped around the neck) and perform the sacramental function? Here comes the analogy: if you believe the devil can possess a human individual, who's the better choice, a priest, or a physician who understands theology and philosophy whose only concern is making the individual whole? (Do you call your wife's divorce attorney for advice? I hope not. You need your own lawyer.) Exorcisms require a disinterested party.

Exorcism is not a normative procedure. It is akin to exterminating rats or lizards from one's home. It is an intervention just as cardiac surgery is. If the priest or rabbi or minister cannot do the job, it is time to call someone else. They probably cannot because they have a vested interested, the perceived will of God. In the author's view a physician trained in psychotherapy is the best choice. Nobody is better than atheist for exorcizing demons. Demons crave respect: no God, no devil, no respect. One does not talk to demons; one poisons them with one's lack of respect. Respect the patient; the demon's most often a "category error". If the demon is real, treat with the patient with sedatives. The demon should be resistant to medication. If the demon had any strength, it would not be hiding in and using some other body. Let it jump into your brain. If you are disciplined, it should find itself in a lethal environment. The physician's lack of theological interest makes the demon very uncomfortable. It could be lethal for the little critter. Seal it and sent it to the pathologists.

In other words, exorcism equals diagnosis and treatment of neurological disease, often very small vascular malformations or malformations in the temporal, frontal, or occipital lobes. The neurosurgeon's ability is most often too blunt an instrument. So much of psychotherapy is neurosurgery performed without touching the patient. It is hard. It often fails because the concept is taken as a futile enterprise. How does the mind and compartment of the therapist change the brain of the patient? Practice, prudence, and indifference to frequent failure are the keys. It takes the temporal and theological virtues. Remember, the physician is not in the miracle business; his enterprise is helping carrying the cross.

There no drugs that remit sins; pharmacotherapy is sometimes adjunctive, ancillary, or worthless. There is no place for the placebo game in neurology. Remember, we cannot treat comportment or minds directly; doctors treat brains.

If someone wants to alter demographics: money, love, a better job, another child, divorce. That often works. Things get better or worse with changes in one's social condition. But we seek some certainty. It seems to me that the preachers who from the Middle

Ages to the Enlightenment took care of the psychotic have quit. Where are the public burnings, the ships of fools, and the cities within cities that shielded the "normal Christian" from the mad? Exorcism was quickly seen to be less effective than the New Testament indicates. Unlike the other sacraments, Penance (without violence) required both intelligence and craft. It was apparent to the most casual observer that the cleric was in general ill-suited to this business of complicated sins and strange perceptions. The same could be said of the typical physician. Some, of course, studied mankind in society and learned a few tricks. Osler and Peabody wrote of these techniques. Freud, Adler, Jung, and Rogers taken together managed to develop a number of techniques which lead to a myriad of others to continue their work.

Unfortunately, psychiatry got too involved in political questions. To his great credit, Freud speculated about society and politics but stuck to the one patient—one doctor paradigm. If you are a physician working for the state, you have picked your poison. This sort of doctor is outside the paradigm. To use a legal analogy, such persons are the defense and the prosecuting attorney, judge and jailer. The patient (client) has a right to separate, independent, and competent physicians. This does not happen. I find both forensic medicine and psychiatry to be arms of the overweening state: different species *Homo legale, NOT Homo medicus.* This is also true about most of public health creatures. The physician is charged with keeping his mouth closed. The amount of collateral damage these public health officers do is not factored into any model of disease detection. They may track the red snapper of tuberculosis with success and little damage.

But the blood–borne and the sexual transmitted disease are another story. How many cures come with divorce attached? The truth may save your life; however, setting you free of guilt, recrimination and enmity is important as well. More attention to the social debris left by these investigations is warranted. These public medical gossips are proof of St James' notion that the tongue is the most dangerous part of the body (*James, chap. 3*). Treat, don't talk. If the physician is competent, the patient's treatment is private. Newspapers are for fishmongers, not gossip mongers. Personal medical information should be reserved for medical files locked in dark places.

Now we have tied the two strands together. First we introduced the inadequacy of the clergy in lifting guilt. Then we presented the physician as the agent of the state. Both try to do things best done in isolation in the middle of the village square at noon. Surgeons rarely operate in the middle of basketball courts. Medicine, including psychotherapy, is best done in clean, will-lighted, and locked rooms.

GETTING SMART

I have no intention of playing Butler's game where sins are illnesses and diseases sins. (*Erewhon*, 1872). The rest of his early affection for and later criticism of Darwin is a road to nowhere. Christ is correct. He is neither ironic nor sarcastic. He is being absolutely frank; the veil drops for a moment. He puts down the challenge that the normative statement always implies. Does the speaker have any positive evidence? In this case, the figure of God lays down the challenge to any other party: do what I have done. Can you heal? Can you remit sins? Can medical science do what God promises: universal, definitive healing? Can medical science do it without resorting to normative demands? If man is truly Cartesian, there should be no problem. One specialist for the soul and another for the bulk of the subject should do the job. One toolkit for each part ought to be available. The indivisible man is tougher. It would take a bigger kit. Let us stop being silly. Medicine has to cure more than one malady, erasing smallpox, polio, malaria, halting cancer of the colon, stroke, or myocardial infarction not in the laboratory that is the modern hospital, but in the home. We lack the certainty of chemistry; we depend too much on time, place, and circumstance for medicine to be a science.

Sins are maladies within the brain that reflect real or perceived compartment which violates Divine Law (or cross- cultural taboos). Thoughts cannot be sins. One cannot control one's thoughts, just as one cannot control one's glomerular filtration rate (renal parameter). Moreover, if wishes were horses, even beggars could ride. Certainly, people can plant all kinds of nonsense in the young and fertile brain. This is the origin of the inappropriate alignment of the will (the soul). Such compartment is sinful. The implantation of thoughts and the manipulation of individuals are behaviors and, hence may be sinful. Compartment contrary to the cross-cultural taboos is sinful unless it is compelled by deadly force or unknown to the rational will. Fugue states or acute psychoses are real occurrences which nearly impossible to prove. The most obvious exception is the direct threat of bodily injury.

We need to get back to the patient on the stretcher. Jesus is not here now. The angel Raphael is not here. However, the latter provided the answer before the former asked the question. The physician ignores the theological questions: he binds up the demon and sends him to Egypt; he rubs the fish goo on the old man's eyes. He does the healer's job. He ignores the politics, the religion, even the will of God. When I am called to see someone with a heart attack, I do not consider God's will, predestination, or divine plans. I get him to the hospital as fast and as safely possible. In Tobit, the angel does not spend a lot of words on abstract concepts. He acts. Certainly, he is God's agent; however, his mission is to serve life. Demons, blindness: it's all the same. He is not praying for death; Raphael is working for life. We are neither gods nor angels nor children of some lesser deity nor the product of the coupling of god and human. If you think the sight of some person bleeding to death is real, then you know that both life and death are realities in a real universe. Medicine is the only human activity where the end sometimes justifies the means. It allows the suspension of reason when ritual is more beneficial. Beneficial means lower morbidity and mortality for all the subjects involved within a very small circle. It applies to the mother we see and the child hidden within equally. It applies to the troubled family, individually and, if possible, collectively. The circle's greatest circumference is the family.

Some speak of treatment as shamanic, rational, or scientific. Most of guidelines are merely expert opinions codified. For many things, we are far more shamanic than we care to admit. We have nails for hips and balloons for arteries. But we are not so good at preventing falls or keeping arteries pristine. We are the pound of cure, not the ounce of prevention. We are too ignorant to bother with much metaphysics or social "engineering"; meta-analysis and system theory is useless where no certain body of knowledge. We are applied anthropologists. Our educations are far too narrow for task of healing. In contradiction to mathematics, medicine has a huge vocabulary, replete with words and ideas "full of sound and fury, signifying nothing". Unlike finance, medicine takes too few factors into account. The political climate, a climate of slow or rapid global warming, and an ambiguous entity that may be called the "climate of opinion" buffet the price fluctuations of everything from gold to coffee. What is true of the rest of man's activities is also true in medicine. Things are far more complex than one can imagine.

So is medicine. Medicine has a bloated dictionary and a narrower view of the man and his environment than the typical commodity trader. To getter smart, we need to understand how far we have strayed beyond our limitations in terms of our "medical" knowledge and how narrowly we have viewed the object of our discipline. Here's an extract from this lexicon:

There is disagreement about the very nature of disease. Of course, that's not new. For example, is heroin addiction a disease? How about wife-beating? What about political dissent? (Only a madman would be unhappy in the "workers' paradise" of the Soviet Union.) The problem goes deeper still. The paradigm fails in pathogenesis. What is the etiology of multiple sclerosis? Is breast cancer always a systemic process? There is plenty of data; however, there is no consensus.

All of this makes scientific materialism (also an appropriate name for Marxist metaphysics) rather silly. There is no inevitable progress; there are many things that exist that cannot be measured. Moreover, pragmatism fails because "good" and "useful" are not easy to define in absolute terms. Stick with empirical materialism? Admit medicine's limitations. We can do better.

Meta-analysis gives you "the big picture" because it is a systematic review of a group of studies on the same topic. In a meta-analysis, researchers statistically analyze results from many studies, often totaling thousands of subjects, to draw the most trustworthy conclusions. Garbage in, garbage out: it all depends on the quality of the studies used.

Randomized controlled trials are considered the gold standard. They compare two groups of subjects. Individuals are randomly placed into control or treatment groups. There is less chance of mischief. If done honestly, this is the only reliable type of study. It is valid only in the population studied. (If all subjects are North Americans, there is no reason to believe that the results will apply in China). Here there is plenty of moral hazard. Among the monsters of modern times, only the Nazis frequently applied this method with scientific rigor. Do you want their data? There were these black men in Alabama with the French disease. How much moral hazard equals the positive knowledge of syphilis worth?

Epidemiological studies are basically surveys of a certain population. The investigators select the patients, so there is plenty of room for bias. Perspective studies follow a group for a period of time. Here there is plenty of room for bias as well: tossing out patients, changing statistical methods, altering therapy, and changing external factors. Retrospective studies are completely worthless. Bias and faulty recall of data are inevitable.

"We don't know" is not the same "is not true". "As best as humanly possible" usually means in developed areas (the "first world"), not the "second" [the former Soviet Union, parts of China, portions of India], surely not the third and largest "world". Incidence, prevalence, and number–needed–to-treat (to prevent one undesirable event) are sociological terms; they depend on one's village. All the RNA inhibitors are useless without a wristwatch. Polio vaccines are useless without peace within a given location. Polio is still around for "political" reasons. No one who realizes this can defend the inherent goodness of mankind. The fall of the Berlin wall was begin of the fall of life expectancy in Eastern Europe and north Asia (the second more diffuse Gulag). The spread of tuberculosis westward and the increase in mortality due to alcohol in Eastern Europe are chronicled by "medical gossip mongers", journalists, and sociologists. Not much is being done. Here we hit a metaphoric brick wall. If medicine is so effective, why isn't everybody healthy? This is the scientific rationale for universal health care. If medicine is scientific, then it must be proved effective everywhere. Saying that political, social, or economic factors preclude this demonstration does not excuse its absence. It leaves doubt as to the efficacy of medicine. We know that malaria is not effectively treated with the same drug in every part of the world. A constantly changing accurate global map of standard drug-resistant malaria and tuberculosis is needed. We know that Kaposi's sarcoma is a different clinical entity in those with and without AIDS. There are many other examples. We need to aim for a unified theory of medicine. The theory and proof of everything is not just for physicists. The goal is valid for physicians as well. Protons do not believe differently in Africa or North America. Burkitt's lymphoma does. There must be a scientific reason. We need an explanation for this. A potent argument for universal care is the same agreement used for the particle collider. If some discipline wants to claim that it is a science, it has to be universal. Otherwise, we are back the village shaman with a hierarchy of tribal witchdoctors.

We need to expand the medical curriculum to include the study of society, not to serve the state, but to treat the individual. The state has plenty of armed partisans; the stranger in his own country has the healing angel. How do we know that this angel exists and has attributes? It is not theology (founded by Philo, a contemporary of Christ and the first, the greatest, and the most copied of his trade. Most dogmatic theology in the Jewish and Christian spheres are replications of or footnotes to Philo of Alexandria). The answer to our problems is hidden centuries earlier. Before Socrates, there were others who thought of the questions that perplexed Plato and Aristotle. We need to recall only two of these shadows who have left us with fragments. Neither splendid dialogues nor pedantic treatises were left to us by Heraclitus and Parmenides.

The author will complete his argument with his view of the necessity of uniting these two metaphysics opposites in order to establish a "medical metaphysics". This synthesis may be unsuccessful, but sooner or later, somebody will have to come up a way to replace the Cartesian man.

"You can't put your foot in the same stream twice". In other words, each moment in life is unique. Heraclitus (ca. 535–475 BC) was a pre-Socratic Greek philosopher, a native of Ephesus, Ionia, on the coast of Asia Minor. Of the "crying philosopher", we have only fragments that seem riddles. They are not; they are tautologies. *We both step and do not step in the same rivers. We are and are not.*

All things are in flux. As opposed to Democritus, "the laughing philosopher", who was certain of the atomic structure of the world, Heraclitus had few fixed ideas, and most of these contained contradictions. I call these proto-archetypes. This grieving sage is concerned with normative questions. The *logos* may be *a sort of natural law, God, the Word that is equivalent to the law...*the philosopher isn't ambiguous. He just does not know. He distinguishes between human laws and divine law "of God".

He removes the human sense of justice from his concept of God; i.e., man is not the image of God: "To God all things are fair and good and just, but men hold some things wrong and some right." God's custom has wisdom, but man's does not. Yet both man and God are alien to each other. There is a sea of misconception separating God and man.

Wisdom is "to know the thought by which all things are steered" Even this prudence does not imply that men are or can be wise. Only God is wise. Thus Heraclitus takes the position of urging men to follow God's plan without much of an idea what that divine plan may be. Man is to search for the archetypes. Yet he cannot know true from false, divine from mundane. Man can strive but can never know the product of his efforts. Again Hippocrates: life is fleeting; the art is long. The physician must withstand both change and ambiguity.

Parmenides, who lived during early 5th century BC, was a philosopher born in Elea, a Greek city on the southern coast of Italy. The single known work of Parmenides is a poem *On Nature* which has survived only in fragments. Approximately 150 lines of the poem remain today; reportedly the original text had 3,000 lines.

In this poem, Parmenides describes two views of reality. In "The Way of Truth" (a part of the poem), he explains how reality is one, change is impossible, and existence is timeless, uniform, and unchanging. This section seems true if one does not consider history. History exists: it is the only constant, and it concerns passages from one object to another. History may speak of kings or species or decay of cities. Reality is one passage after another. The concept of History refutes Parmenides' first thesis. In "The Way of Opinion", he explains the world of appearances, which is false and deceitful. The individual life is small and transient; however, the craft of understanding is hard and is built on constant revision of opinions. If the appearance deceives, the physician must attempt to come to some conclusion about the object in question (disease, patient, behavior). In the alternative:

Helplessness guides the wandering thought in their breasts; they are carried along deaf and blind alike, dazed, beasts without judgment, convinced that to be and not to be are the same and not the same, and that the road of all things is a backward-turning one. (B 6.5-9)

You must debar your thought from this way of search, nor let ordinary experience in its variety force you along this way, (namely, that of allowing) the eye, sightless as it is, and the ear, full of sound, and the tongue, to rule; but (you must) judge by means of the Reason (Logos) the much-contested proof which is expounded.. (B 7.1-8.2)

The structure of the cosmos is a fundamental binary principle that governs the manifestations of all the particulars, says Parmenides. This author disagrees. There is but one a cycle of day and night, a body inseparable its soul (perhaps until death). Parmenides states:

The mortals lay down and decided well to name two forms (i.e. the flaming light and obscure darkness of night), out of which it is necessary not to make one, and in this they are led astray. (B 8.53-4)

He is wrong. The error is not seeing both as part of one indivisible being. THERE IS NO DUALITY, ONLY UNITY. Appearances are deceptive because the changing mask of the unitary being. Parmenides is on target when he writes:

Thinking and the thought that it is are the same; for you will not find thought apart from what is, in relation to which it is uttered. (B 8.34-36)

This is the same thing that St. Anselm tells and the very opposite of Peirce's declaration. This statement is the foundation of Platonic, Christian, Jewish, and Muslim metaphysics. St. Anselm and Parmenides are speaking of the common cross-cultural archetypes (the night world). Peirce and

Aristotle speak of the common reality (the day world). Plato explains unity of these phases in his famous analogy of the cave. The strange shadows and statues of Plato's cave are the archetypes and paradigms of God (or the cross-cultural Unconscious). The *logos* of Heraclitus is not the *logos* of theology, but it is the foundation upon the theologian and physician may explain the flux of *all things* while maintaining the transcendental constants which govern the flux of *all things*. Ryle, Peirce, and Aristotle speak of the day; Plato and Jung speak of the night. Aquinas, Spinoza, and Kant speak of both. Both are the province of the true physician.

There seems to be another world, a place of darkness, which is unique to each individual, and it is the world of dreams, souls, minds…. Its elements are common to all just as the reality of the day is, but the night world is arranged differently and is most often a secret to the individual himself. How does one (the patient) discover the sickness within this dark world? By contrast, the order of the day world is obvious. Recall appearance deceive us; the world is one. The universe is singular. In dormitories the sick and injured slept. Aesculapius' disciples knew the answer to this enigma. NOT TWO WORLDS BUT TWO HEMISPHERES OF THE SAME WORLD:

More than a thousand years before Jesus was born, the cult grew very popular. The healing temple was called an asclepieion; pilgrims flocked to them to be healed. They slept overnight and reported their dreams to a priest the following day. He prescribed a cure, often a visit to the baths or a gymnasium. There seems another world, a place of darkness, which is unique to each individual, and it is the world of dreams, souls, and minds all within the indivisible person. The temple's priests knew their "geography" and understood its importance. In the uncertainty of Heraclitus, there remained only one certainty: the finite individual longing for that which infinite: life, knowledge, contentment. Health was and remains the integrated person. Sickness is decay, damage, and disassociation within the person.

People accept knowledge only when it is effective and safe. Allopathic medicine has fallen into the two traps that have snared religion and science; it is doubly cursed. Medicine is ineffective relative to its claims and at the same time dangerous. Patients have not a bit of interest in whether therapy is shamanic, rational, empirical, and/or scientific. They want safe and effective therapies delivered with compassion. In cases where there is no reliable therapy, the patient, unencumbered by financial or geographical constraints, realizes that he is being hoodwinked. High prices, fancy machines, or arrogant physicians do not disguise inadequate therapy.

This is what Aesculapius knew at the start. This was the knowledge that caused the lord of the sky to condemn him. This is the knowledge that brought him glory after death. Like the first psychoanalysts, the priests of Aesculapius knew the value of dreams. But we are a long way from where the art started. We have lost much along the way. We have bartered and bargained away much of our profession's treasure for other precious things. Only time will tell if these transactions were profitable. I doubt that they were. We have reached a plateau on which we are marooned. The uncommon triumph of "modern medicine" will remain. Churches will pronounced the word "miracle" far too often. Our present knowledge will certainly increase; however, it will no good for the poor and powerless. We are Darwinian; we have reached beyond genetics to achieve the triumph of demographics. The rich are stronger than poor because they have food. They have schools. Soldiers rarely come and massacre them. Money, political differences, and economic injustice have tripped up "scientific medicine". Science should be indifferent to these factors. Medicine isn't. Moreover, our understanding of the brain is so lacking that we do not realize that the present medications are no more than ancillary therapy which allows (when given in minimal doses) to engage the patient in psychotherapy. (Please my other works for an elaboration of this argument.) We conclude with a bitter pill.

"In the end the words were said by Oliver Cromwell: "I beseech you, in the bowels of Christ; think it possible you may be mistaken"... I owe it as a human being ... to stand by here by the pond as a survivor and witness. We have to cure ourselves of the itch for absolute knowledge and power."

These are the words of Jacob Bronowski (from *The Ascent of Man* page 374, 1973, Little, Brown, Boston). The pond is within the confines of Auschwitz. We cannot afford to remedy the "itch" for knowledge; we are surrounded by ignorance.

Bronowski was standing in the midst of the consequence of the coupling of pride and ignorance. We need to cure our impulse for power before that power eradicates the human parasite from the planet. I don't agree with Bronowski about the "itch" for knowledge. There is a paucity of knowledge, a scarcity of virtue, and a virtual absence of good. They are acquired in this sequence. To repeat, Euclid reminded one of the Ptolemaic pharaohs that "there is no royal road to understanding geometry". Nor is there a safe, smooth path to achieving the paradigm of the truly good physician. There are, however, many traps and obstacles; many charlatans and thieves; "many purveyors of the culture of death".

It matters little in this context whether God or Redemption exist. Physicians are still vivisecting man into body and mind, neglecting the soul. The author believes God exists and acts in the world. However, God cannot open the ears or tear off the eyelids of those who eschew knowledge or mistake it for technical expertise.

The book is about the healing angel, Raphael. This the angel who came as a friend, worked with prudence and discretion, treating the human as both a material and spiritual being. This is the angel who converted prayers for death to praises for life in a land where his patients were a tiny and persecuted minority.

It is the physician's task to help the patient make this selection. Yet, we are frail, oppressed by government and economic reality over which we have no control. I have suggested ways to turn aside these challenges. Life is brief. Temptation is ever nipping at our heels. It is a hard craft, this medicine. It calls the physician to become the silent and hidden servant. Our teachers are fools. We age, and our brains exhaust themselves. For those of us addicted to medicine, it is a bitter existence. We suffer from uncertainty, from not having the necessary knowledge, from having the certainty of defeat beside us. Death is our shadow. We are still painfully frail and profound in our ignorance.

APPENDICES

Appendix I: Aquinas and system builders

St. Thomas is the greatest of the modified realists. He is the theologian for Christians of all stripes, Jews, and Muslims. The reason for this is simple; he took everything he could fit into the *Summa Theologica* (often word–for-word) from Islamic and Hebrew sources as well the Church fathers who happened to fit into his system. His great work is a summation of Christian belief defended by every relevant Jewish and Islamic source. He examined the ancients through the perspective of three medieval faiths. Like Plato, Aristotle, Spinoza, and Kant, he is a system-builder. Aquinas, along with Plato and Spinoza began with metaphysics. Aristotle had his metaphysics expanded by many who used his work as a foundation. Kant's work was pushed to its inevitable conclusion by Fitche who was the bridge between Kant's rationalism and Hegel's fanciful idealism. Here are the names of the seven gifts of the Holy Spirit along with a description of each gift, as defined by St. Thomas Aquinas (taken from a standard reference which confirms to the teaching of Roman Church)

Wisdom - The gift of wisdom perfects a person's speculative reason in matters of judgment about the truth.

Knowledge - The gift of knowledge perfects a person's practical reason in matters of judgment about the truth.

Judgment - The gift of counsel perfects a person's practical reason in the apprehension of truth and allows the person to respond prudently.

Courage -The gift of Courage allows people the firmness of mind [that] is required both in doing good and in enduring evil, especially with regard to goods or evils that are difficult [to tolerate].

Understanding - Also called "Common Sense." The gift of understanding perfects a person's speculative reason in the apprehension of truth. It is the gift whereby self-evident principles are known

Piety - Piety is the gift whereby, at the Holy Spirit's instigation, we pay worship and duty to God as our Father.

Fear of the Lord - This gift is described by Aquinas as a fear of separating oneself from God. He describes the gift as a "filial fear," like a child's fear of offending his father, rather than a "servile fear," that is, a fear of punishment.

Aquinas says the first four of these gifts (wisdom, understanding, knowledge, and counsel) direct the intellect, while the other three gifts (fortitude, piety, and fear of the Lord) direct the will toward God.

from "http://en.wikipedia.org/wiki/Seven_gifts_of_the_Holy_Spirit

In some respects, the gifts are similar to the virtues but a key distinction is that the virtues operate under the impetus of human reason (prompted by grace), whereas the gifts operate under the impetus of the Holy Spirit; the former can be used when one wishes, but the latter operate only when the Holy Spirit wishes. The former are like the oars of a boat; the latter, the sails. The reader will note that I disagree entirely with this view. For me there are only oars which are hard to fabricate. The Holy Spirit is a network of lighthouses. One needs to row to the shore marked by the beacons.

Dante based his *Comedia* on Thomas' thought. The most controversial concept within *Paradiso* is this concept: the greater the intellect, passion, and will (the components of the soul) of the blessed, the closer to God the "saved" are placed. It's simple addition; higher sums merit higher places. This is true until one reaches the higher spheres of paradise where dogmatic (archetypical) considerations become dominant.

It is also quite clear that the Cartesian man did not originate with Descartes. He was around long before and long after Aquinas; it is my view that it is time that he exit the stage. Shakespeare and Cervantes found no way to divide body, mind, and soul. That crazy Spanish knight with his faithful squire dismissed both Nominalism and the Cartesian separation with pathos and blinding insight. The perplexing Danish prince, that Scottish murderer with the dagger of the mind always before him, and that wagering Jew among many others fretting before an often indifferent public did not allow an easy dissection of mind, soul, and body.

A major task of the theologian is to champion modified realism in the age of the indivisible individual. Alfred Adler called his theory individual psychology because the single person was indivisible. However, we are physicians. We are not theologians; we are interested in that human specimen that cannot be divided. The theologian and the physician have plenty of work before them. There is no reason not to let them to compete; there are plenty of problems to be solved. Some rugged competition might wake them both up to the reality of human suffering.

Here we need to make obvious two implied rejections and one radical and extreme affirmation. We are in the "doctoring craft". Despite the brilliance of Ludwig Binswanger and his perfection of the clinical biography, the author rejects completely his philosophical foundations which seem unnecessary baggage. The Binswanger method needs greater application throughout medicine. It is especially useful for difficult diagnoses.

Nothing from Husserl or Heidegger need concern us. We practice medicine; we have no interest in Binswanger's superior plane (plateau) of existence. Nor does the author accept the primacy of form over content championed by Jaspers. The second more subtle rejection is that of the work of Noam Chomsky (particularly *Cartesian Linguistics)* and Jerry Fodor. The author embraces Ryle: We cannot be certain of what is going within own or another's body (including the brain). We cannot be certain of our own minds nor can we "read" the minds of others. We are individuals living in villages who know little of our place in the great map of the world. We know the world by following rules (regulations concerning language, logic, scientific validity). The other sources of "knowing things" are archetypes (outside of rational thought and morality) and distinct moral paradigms which we learn, which are external to ourselves. Medicine is concerned with only two non-medical archetypes:

1. The treatment of the dead (see *Antigone*);

2. Cardinal Newman's statement that we are the property of a unique Deity

a. because He has created us

b. because He has revealed special knowledge to mankind,

c. because He has a contract with us,

d. because He has "paid" for our sins (violations of his laws). This applies to all men whether Christian or not. Any one (or more) of these clauses is sufficient. There are other archetypical rules which do not concern us. We will not pursue any others.

Appendix II: The Fall of Hippocrates:

Hippocratic medicine was humble and passive. The therapeutic approach was based on "the healing power of nature" ("vis medicatrix naturae"). According to this doctrine, the body contains within itself the power to re-balance the four humors and heal itself. Hippocrates was reluctant to administer drugs and engage in specialized treatment that might prove to be wrongly chosen; generalized therapy followed a generalized diagnosis. Hippocratic medicine was notable for its strict professionalism, discipline and rigorous practice. The Hippocratic School gave importance to the clinical doctrines of observation and documentation. These doctrines dictate that physicians record their findings and their medicinal methods in a very clear and objective manner, so that these records may be passed down and employed by other physicians. Hippocrates made careful, regular note of many symptoms including complexion, pulse, fever, pains, movement, and excretions. Hippocrates began to categorize illnesses as acute, chronic, endemic and epidemic, and use particular terms: exacerbation, relapse, resolution, crisis, paroxysm, peak, and convalescence. Ancient Greek schools of medicine were split into the Knidian and Koan. The Knidian school of medicine focused on diagnosis and was dependent on many false assumptions about the human body. The Knidian School consequently failed to distinguish when one disease manifested variations of in the order and degree of symptoms The Hippocratic School or Koan school achieved greater success by applying general diagnoses and passive treatments. The serious observer with a gentle, but inquisitive disposition was the clinical model until the last gasp of the Western European supremacy (August, 1914).

Galen was the surgeon to gladiators, the "cutter" of Barbary apes, thus the patron saint of vivisection. He was a shameless self-promoter; he would be at home in the contemporary medical environment. Hippocrates touched only to search the body's surface and with great gentleness. He was the servant of his craft; he kept secrets. He was listening, watching, and recording. Until two hundred years ago, he represented the epitome of his profession: no longer. Ironic: Galen is of the present. Five hundred years after falling to a Flemish anatomist's dissections, he is back. Bernard, Virchow, and all those painless, antiseptic surgeons have pushed him back into the limelight. It is Hippocrates who is stuck like a beetle in amber.

www.ingramcontent.com/pod-product-compliance
Lightning Source LLC
Chambersburg PA
CBHW070859180526
45168CB00005B/1873